This Journal Belongs to:

_____

If lost, please contact:

_____

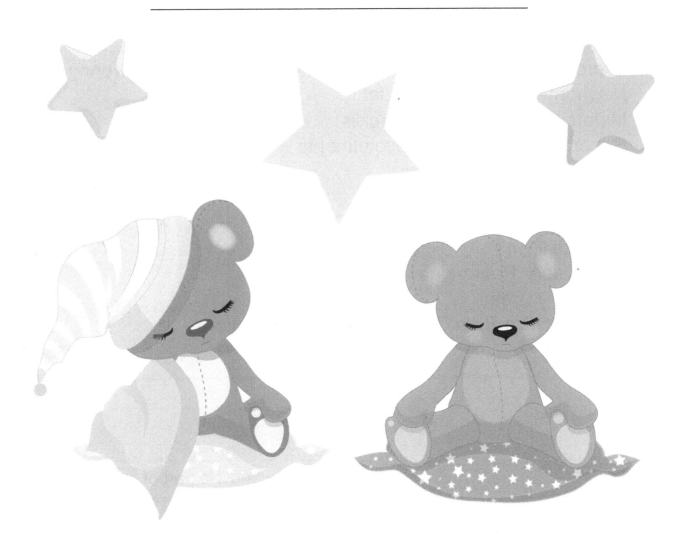

You're expecting! Here's what you can expect in this Pregnancy journal:

This is such an exciting time in your life! This journal will allow you to revisit your pregnancy in years to come! Be sure to scan the whole journal right away so you know where to find everything described below, so that you can get the most out of it.

- Pregnancy Journal Pages to record when you first found out you were pregnant plus Weeks 4 – 41 (just in case you're overdue!)
- 3 journal pages to summarize each of your trimesters
- Space for My First Love Letter to My Baby
- Space for listing your Baby Name Ideas
- Growing a Healthy Baby Meal Planner
- Foods/Drinks to Avoid & Ones to Add to Your Shopping List
- Exercise During Pregnancy – Questions that Need Answering
- Newborn Baby Shopping List
- Maternity Hospital Bag Checklist
- Record of My Prenatal Appointments
- My Baby Shower
- My Sonogram Photos
- My Fetal Movements Tracking Charts
- My Birth Plan
- My Nursery Room Ideas
- My Family Tree
- Important Pre-Birth Questions & Considerations
- The Birth

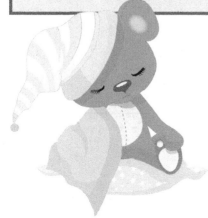

I am Pregnant!

Date I found out: _____

How far along was I?: _____

How I found out: _____

My Estimated Due Date:

_____

_____

_____

My reaction: _____

_____

_____

_____

Did I suspect I was pregnant?: _____

_____

_____

_____

Who I first told that I was pregnant & his/her reaction: _____

_____

_____

_____

What else do I remember about the day I found out that I was pregnant?: _____

_____

_____

_____

_____

_____

_____

_____

Baby Name Ideas

Girl's Names

Boy's Names

Other thoughts:

My First Love Letter to My Unborn Baby

Newborn Baby Shopping Checklist

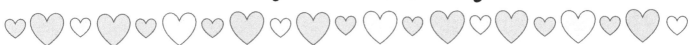

TIP: Keep in mind that baby grows quickly so don't buy too many clothes or diapers of the same size before baby is born. Don't forget to sign up for prenatal classes and Baby CPR classes.

Clothing

- [ ] Onesies
- [ ] Sleepwear
- [ ] Undershirts
- [ ] Socks
- [ ] Slippers
- [ ] Pants or shorts
- [ ] Shirts
- [ ] Dresses
- [ ] Scratch prevention mittens
- [ ] Baby hat
- [ ] Sweaters and jackets for babies born in cool weather
- [ ] Snowsuit & mitts for baby born in winter

Sleeping

- [ ] Crib & mattress
- [ ] Sheets for crib
- [ ] Baby monitor
- [ ] Swaddling blankets
- [ ] Baby sling
- [ ]
- [ ]

Bathing

- [ ] Baby wash cloths
- [ ] Baby hooded towels
- [ ] Soft-bristled baby brush
- [ ] Baby body wash/shampoo
- [ ] Baby lotion
- [ ] Baby bathtub
- [ ]
- [ ]
- [ ]

Diapering

- [ ] Diaper rash ointment
- [ ] Diaper pad &/or change table
- [ ] Baby wipes
- [ ] Diapers
- [ ] Diaper pail
- [ ] Diaper bag
- [ ]
- [ ]
- [ ]
- [ ]

Feeding

- [ ] Formula
- [ ] Baby bottles, bottle liners, bottle brush
- [ ] Nipple cream
- [ ] Breast pump & milk storage bags
- [ ] Nursing pillow
- [ ] Burp cloths & receiving blankets
- [ ] Nursing bras & pads
- [ ] Bibs
- [ ] High chair

Miscellaneous

- [ ] Baby laundry detergent
- [ ] Infant car seat
- [ ] Stroller
- [ ] Baby thermometer
- [ ] Mobile for crib
- [ ] Rocking chair
- [ ] Night light
- [ ] Nasal bulb syringe
- [ ] Nail scissors
- [ ] Pacifiers
- [ ] Baby swing

My Pregnancy Journal

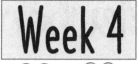

My Baby Bump

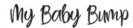

My baby is the size of a poppy seed.

My Weight:

My Belly Circumference:

How I've Been Feeling:

What I want to remember most about this week:

My Pregnancy Journal

My Baby Bump

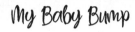

My baby is the size of a sesame seed.

My Weight:

My Belly Circumference:

How I've Been Feeling:

My baby's tissues & organ systems begin to develop in Week 5.

What I want to remember most about this week:

My Pregnancy Journal

My Baby Bump

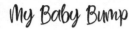

My baby is the size of a lentil, approx. ¼".

My Weight:

My Belly Circumference:

How I've Been Feeling:

The neural tube in baby's back closes, heart & other organs are developing, small arm buds appear, & eyes & ears primitively form.

What I want to remember most about this week:

My Pregnancy Journal

My Baby Bump

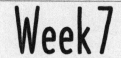

My baby has doubled in size since last week, and is now the size of a blueberry.

My Weight:

My Belly Circumference:

How I've Been Feeling:

My baby's brain & head are growing, nostrils and retinas are starting to develop, leg buds appear, & the arm buds look like paddles.

What I want to remember most about this week:

My Pregnancy Journal

My Baby Bump

My baby is the size of a kidney bean, and over ½" long.

My Weight:

My Belly Circumference:

How I've Been Feeling:

Fingers and nose are forming, and the leg buds look like paddles.

What I want to remember most about this week:

My Pregnancy Journal

My Baby Bump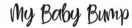

My baby is the size of a grape. The eyes are fully formed, but closed.

My Weight:

My Belly Circumference:

How I've Been Feeling:

Baby's eyelids form, baby's arms grow, elbows appear, & toes are developing.

What I want to remember most about this week:

My Pregnancy Journal

My baby is the size of a kumquat, measures a bit over 1" from head to buttocks..

My Baby Bump

My Weight:

My Belly Circumference:

How I've Been Feeling:

My baby can bend the elbows, the toes & fingers aren't as webbed in appearance as they get longer, and the head gets rounder.

What I want to remember most about this week:

My Pregnancy Journal

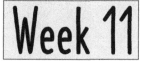

My Baby Bump

My baby is the size of a fig, over
1.5" long, & can kick & stretch..

My Weight:

My Belly
Circumference:

How I've Been Feeling:

Baby is inhaling & exhaling small amounts of amniotic fluid, exercising the lungs.

What I want to remember most about this week:

My Pregnancy Journal

My Baby Bump

My baby is the size of a lime, and is over 2" long from head to baby's butt.

My Weight:

My Belly Circumference:

How I've Been Feeling:

Baby's muscles are getting bigger, & baby is opening & closing his/her fingers, and kicking his/her arms and legs.

What I want to remember most about this week:

My First Trimester

What I enjoyed most & least about the first trimester

How I Felt This Trimester

My Favorite Memories

My Pregnancy Journal

My Baby Bump

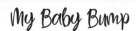

My baby is the size of a pea pod, approx. 3" long, & weighs 1 oz..

My Weight:

My Belly Circumference:

How I've Been Feeling:

Baby's body is catching up to the growth of his head. All essential organs & body systems have developed, baby's kidneys are working, testicles & ovaries are formed, fingerprints are starting.

What I want to remember most about this week:

My Pregnancy Journal

My baby is the size of a lemon, 3.5" long,
& can make some facial expressions.

My Baby Bump

My Weight:

My Belly Circumference:

How I've Been Feeling:

Your baby exhibits sucking reflexes, and is growing fine-like hair (lanugo) to help regulate his/her temperature.

What I want to remember most about this week:

My Pregnancy Journal

My Baby Bump

My baby is the size of an apple, 4" long, & 2.5 oz..

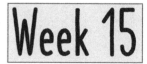

My Weight:

My Belly Circumference:

How I've Been Feeling:

Baby's bones are hardening, muscles continue to form, & baby's closed eyes are starting to be sensitive to light.

What I want to remember most about this week:

My Pregnancy Journal

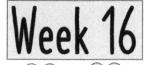

Week 16

My Baby Bump

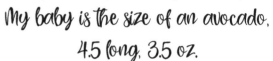

My baby is the size of an avocado, 4.5 long, 3.5 oz.

My Weight:

My Belly Circumference:

How I've Been Feeling:

Baby's heart is pumping around 49 pints (28 L) of blood around his/her body every day!

What I want to remember most about this week:

My Pregnancy Journal

My Baby Bump

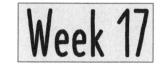

My baby is the size of a turnip, weighs 5 oz, & is 5" long..

My Weight:

My Belly Circumference:

How I've Been Feeling:

Baby's hearing is pretty good, & can hear your muffled voice & music. Your baby has his own set of distinct fingerprints.

What I want to remember most about this week:

My Pregnancy Journal

Week 18

My Baby Bump

My baby is the size of a bell pepper, weighs 7 oz, & is 5.5 long..

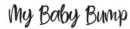

My Weight:

My Belly Circumference:

How I've Been Feeling:

Your baby is growing eyebrows.

What I want to remember most about this week:

My Pregnancy Journal

My Baby Bump

My baby is the size of a large tomato, weighs 8.5 oz, & is 6" long.

My Weight:

My Belly Circumference:

How I've Been Feeling:

Hair may be beginning to grow on your baby's head, the brain is specializing, & you may be feeling your baby's movements at this point.

What I want to remember most about this week:

My Pregnancy Journal

My Baby Bump

My baby is the size of a banana, & is 6.5" from head to butt or 10" to the heels.

My Weight:

My Belly Circumference:

How I've Been Feeling:

You are halfway through your pregnancy! Your baby is moving a lot within your womb now.

What I want to remember most about this week:

My Pregnancy Journal

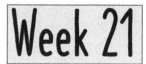

My Baby Bump

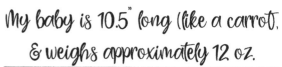
My baby is 10.5" long (like a carrot),
& weighs approximately 12 oz.

My Weight:

My Belly
Circumference:

How I've Been Feeling:

If you are feeling your baby's movements, you will begin to recognize periods of wakefulness and sleeping. Baby's eyes move rapidly under the eyelids.

What I want to remember most about this week:

My Pregnancy Journal

My baby is the size of a spaghetti squash, weighs 1 lb, & is 11" long from head to butt.

My Baby Bump

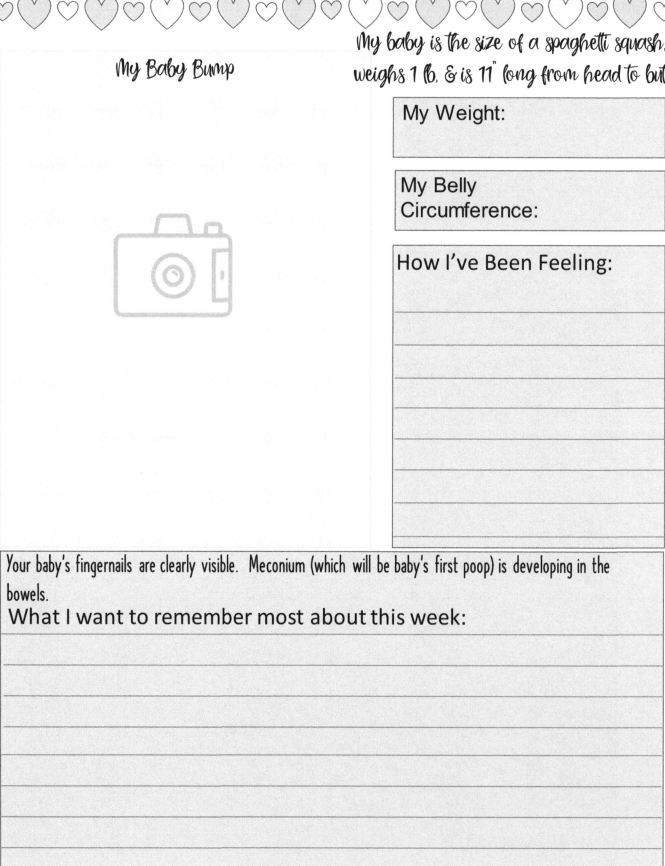

My Weight:

My Belly Circumference:

How I've Been Feeling:

Your baby's fingernails are clearly visible. Meconium (which will be baby's first poop) is developing in the bowels.

What I want to remember most about this week:

My Pregnancy Journal

My Baby Bump

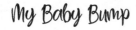

My baby is the size of a large mango.

My Weight:

My Belly Circumference:

How I've Been Feeling:

Your baby's hearing is improving to hear other sounds outside of the womb.

What I want to remember most about this week:

My Pregnancy Journal

My Baby Bump

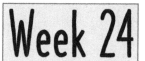

My baby is about 12" (30 cm) long, & weighs 1 ¼ lb.

My Weight:

My Belly Circumference:

How I've Been Feeling:

Your baby is considered possibly "viable" if he is born now, but really needs more time to grow & maximize the chances for survival outside the womb. Your baby makes facial expressions.

What I want to remember most about this week:

My Pregnancy Journal

My Baby Bump

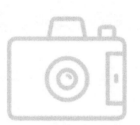

My baby is the size of a rutabaga. It is about 13.5" in length, & 1 ½ lb.

My Weight:

My Belly Circumference:

How I've Been Feeling:

Your baby is putting on more fat in preparation for birth.

What I want to remember most about this week:

My Pregnancy Journal

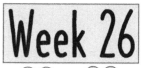

My Baby Bump

My baby is 14" long, 1 & 2/3 lb.

My Weight:

My Belly Circumference:

How I've Been Feeling:

Your baby can likely recognize your voice & that of your partner. Baby's tastebuds are developed. The lungs continue to develop.

What I want to remember most about this week:

My Pregnancy Journal

My Baby Bump

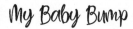

My baby is the size of a cauliflower, is 14.5 long, & 2 lb in weight.

My Weight:

My Belly Circumference:

How I've Been Feeling:

You may feel when your baby hiccups. Your baby is also experiencing more regular patterns of sleep and wakefulness, which you may start to notice.

What I want to remember most about this week:

My Pregnancy Journal

My Baby Bump

My baby is the size of an eggplant, weighs 2 ¼ lb., & is 15" long.

My Weight:

My Belly Circumference:

How I've Been Feeling:

Your baby's eyes now open & close, have eyelashes, & can form tears. The irises are now pigmented.

What I want to remember most about this week:

My Second Trimester

What I enjoyed most & least about the second trimester

_____
_____
_____
_____
_____
_____
_____
_____

How I Felt This Trimester

_____
_____
_____
_____
_____

My Favorite Memories

_____
_____
_____
_____
_____
_____

My Pregnancy Journal

My Baby Bump

My baby is the size of a butternut squash, 15" long, & 2.5 lb.

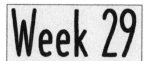

My Weight:

My Belly Circumference:

How I've Been Feeling:

Your baby's brain continues to develop the neurons needed for intelligence & personality.

What I want to remember most about this week:

My Pregnancy Journal

My Baby Bump

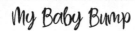

My baby is the size of a big cabbage, weighs 3 lb. & is 15 ¾" long.

My Weight:

My Belly Circumference:

How I've Been Feeling:

Try shining a flashlight on your belly, & you may notice your baby move or kick.

What I want to remember most about this week:

My Pregnancy Journal

My Baby Bump

My baby is the weight of a coconut.

My Weight:

My Belly Circumference:

How I've Been Feeling:

Your baby is getting longer & bigger, so he/she takes on the curled-up, fetal position in utero until birth now.

What I want to remember most about this week:

My Pregnancy Journal

Week 32

My Baby Bump

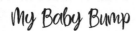

My baby is 16 ¾" long, & weighs approx. 3 ¾ lb..

My Weight:

My Belly Circumference:

How I've Been Feeling:

If born now, your baby has a good chance of surviving & being healthy, although baby's lungs aren't fully developed yet.

What I want to remember most about this week:

My Pregnancy Journal

My Baby Bump

My baby is the weight of a pineapple, weighs 4 lb, & is 17" long..

My Weight:

My Belly Circumference:

How I've Been Feeling:

You may notice that your baby's activity level & responses are dependent on your own actions, such as whether you've just eaten or you're in a noisy environment.

What I want to remember most about this week:

My Pregnancy Journal

My Baby Bump

My baby is 18" long, & 4 ¾ lb.

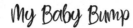

My Weight:

My Belly Circumference:

How I've Been Feeling:

This is a great time to sing lullabies to your baby, as baby is more likely to recognize them after birth.

What I want to remember most about this week:

My Pregnancy Journal

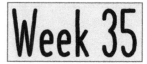

My Baby Bump

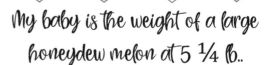
My baby is the weight of a large honeydew melon at 5 ¼ lb..

My Weight:

My Belly Circumference:

How I've Been Feeling:

The amniotic fluid surrounding baby is decreasing. 97% of babies are head-down at this point, in preparation for the birth.

What I want to remember most about this week:

My Pregnancy Journal

My Baby Bump

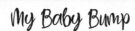

My baby is 18.5" long, & weighs close to 6 lb.

My Weight:

My Belly Circumference:

How I've Been Feeling:

Baby is shedding the lanugo hair & vernix caseosa (white waxy substance) this week. Baby's sucking is fully developed now.

What I want to remember most about this week:

My Pregnancy Journal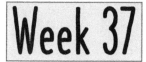

My Baby Bump

My baby is approximately 19" long, & 6 1/3 lb.

My Weight:

My Belly Circumference:

How I've Been Feeling:

You pass antibodies to your baby through the umbilical cord. Baby's grasp is improving, ready to grasp your fingers (and heart) when born.

What I want to remember most about this week:

My Pregnancy Journal

My Baby Bump

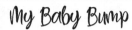

My baby weighs about 7 lb, & is 19.5" long.

My Weight:

My Belly Circumference:

How I've Been Feeling:

Baby continues to improve his/her breathing, circulation, & digestion.

What I want to remember most about this week:

My Pregnancy Journal

My Baby Bump

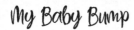

My baby is the weight of a watermelon, around 7 lb.

My Weight:

My Belly Circumference:

How I've Been Feeling:

If you haven't given birth yet, baby is ready to meet you any day now!

What I want to remember most about this week:

My Pregnancy Journal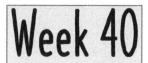

My Baby Bump

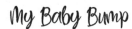

My baby is the size of a pumpkin, weighs approx. 7.5 lb, & 20" long.

My Weight:

My Belly
Circumference:

How I've Been Feeling:

Your baby will be born with many natural reflexes necessary for survival (rooting for the nipple, suckling, etc.)

What I want to remember most about this week:

My Pregnancy Journal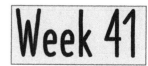

My Baby Bump

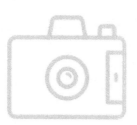

My Weight:

My Belly Circumference:

How I've Been Feeling:

It should be any time now! Enjoy the last few days of your pregnancy. You'll miss feeling the baby's movements in your womb after birth.

What I want to remember most about this week:

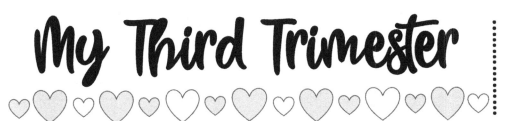

My Third Trimester

Weeks 29-40ish

What I enjoyed most & least about the third trimester

How I Felt This Trimester

My Favorite Memories

Foods/Drinks to Avoid on Shopping List

FISH, MEATS, & EGGS

Avoid raw, undercooked or smoked meat, chicken, fish and shellfish, including sushi, oysters, and clams. Deli meats should be limited, & only eaten when cooked to kill potential bacteria. Liver and other organ meats are high in Vitamin A – consult with a dietician or your doctor before consuming too much during pregnancy. Also limit how often you eat tuna, salmon, & swordfish (higher mercury content). Avoid raw eggs & foods that contain them (raw cookie/cake batter, eggnog, etc.).

DAIRY

Avoid unpasteurised milk (be sure you drink pasteurised milk), soft cheeses such as blue cheese, feta, brie, and several other kinds of these soft cheeses. Be sure to research the kinds that are and aren't safe.

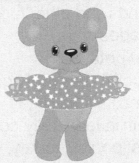

VEGGIES & FRUIT

Wash them all very well. Cook them, whenever possible. Raw sprouts (alfalfa, clover, radish, & bean sprouts) are a concern. Avoid bruised veggies & fruit, as bacteria may have invaded the damaged areas. Also avoid unripe papaya, which has similar effects to oxytocin, which stimulates labor.

MISCELLANEOUS

Speak to your doctor about which medications are safe/not safe. Be careful of herbal remedies – speak to your doctor first as many are unsafe during pregnancy. Avoid all alcohol & drugs. Avoid artificial sweeteners, limit caffeine intake, soda, and other fatty or high-calorie foods with no nutritional value. Avoid unpasteurised juices too. Avoid foods with excess salt and trans fats.

Disclaimer: This list does **not** include every food item you should avoid. It is up to you to do your research & speak to your healthcare provider if you're not sure.

Foods/Drinks to Add on Shopping List

SOME GOOD IDEAS

- A prenatal vitamin and mineral supplement is recommended. Ensure you are getting enough folate/folic acid for at least 3 months before and at the start of your pregnancy to reduce the risk of neural tube defects.
- Almonds and other mixed nuts
- Avocados
- Sweet potatoes
- Broccoli & dark leafy greens (well washed)
- Protein in lean, fully-cooked meats, poultry, turkey, veal, etc.
- Pasteurised milk
- Hard cheeses like cheddar
- Yogurt
- Cold-pressed olive oil
- Fully-cooked eggs and omelettes
- Oranges

RECIPE I'D LIKE TO TRY

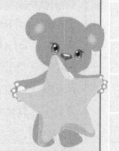

Disclaimer: This list does **not** include every food item you should be including in your diet. It is up to you to do your research & speak to your healthcare provider if you're not sure.

Growing a Healthy Baby Meal Planner

	Breakfast	Lunch	Supper	Snacks
Monday				
Tuesday				
Wednesday				
Thursday				
Friday				
Saturday				
Sunday				

Alternate Healthy Baby Meal Planner

	Breakfast	Lunch	Supper	Snacks
Monday				
Tuesday				
Wednesday				
Thursday				
Friday				
Saturday				
Sunday				

Nursery Room Ideas

Favorite website examples: _____

_____
_____
_____
_____
_____
_____

Color scheme & theme ideas: _____

_____
_____
_____
_____
_____
_____
_____

Draw out the layout, or add more notes:

My Baby Shower

Friends & family who attended:

Games we played:

Baby Shower Photo:

My Favorite Memories of the Day:

My Prenatal Appointments

Date:	Gestational Age:	My Weight Gain:	Blood Pressure:

Other important & memorable events (baby's heartbeat, what doctor said, etc.):

_____

_____

_____

_____

Date:	Gestational Age:	My Weight Gain:	Blood Pressure:

Other important & memorable events (baby's heartbeat, what doctor said, etc.):

_____

_____

_____

_____

Date:	Gestational Age:	My Weight Gain:	Blood Pressure:

Other important & memorable events (baby's heartbeat, what doctor said, etc.):

_____

_____

_____

_____

Date:	Gestational Age:	My Weight Gain:	Blood Pressure:

Other important & memorable events (baby's heartbeat, what doctor said, etc.):

_____

_____

_____

_____

My Prenatal Appointments

Date: _____

Gestational Age: _____

My Weight Gain: _____

Blood Pressure: _____

Other important & memorable events (baby's heartbeat, what doctor said, etc.):

_____

_____

_____

_____

Date: _____

Gestational Age: _____

My Weight Gain: _____

Blood Pressure: _____

Other important & memorable events (baby's heartbeat, what doctor said, etc.):

_____

_____

_____

_____

Date: _____

Gestational Age: _____

My Weight Gain: _____

Blood Pressure: _____

Other important & memorable events (baby's heartbeat, what doctor said, etc.):

_____

_____

_____

_____

Date: _____

Gestational Age: _____

My Weight Gain: _____

Blood Pressure: _____

Other important & memorable events (baby's heartbeat, what doctor said, etc.):

_____

_____

_____

_____

My Prenatal Appointments

Date: _____   Gestational Age: _____   My Weight Gain: _____   Blood Pressure: _____

Other important & memorable events (baby's heartbeat, what doctor said, etc.):

_____
_____
_____
_____

Date: _____   Gestational Age: _____   My Weight Gain: _____   Blood Pressure: _____

Other important & memorable events (baby's heartbeat, what doctor said, etc.):

_____
_____
_____
_____

Date: _____   Gestational Age: _____   My Weight Gain: _____   Blood Pressure: _____

Other important & memorable events (baby's heartbeat, what doctor said, etc.):

_____
_____
_____
_____

Date: _____   Gestational Age: _____   My Weight Gain: _____   Blood Pressure: _____

Other important & memorable events (baby's heartbeat, what doctor said, etc.):

_____
_____
_____
_____

My Prenatal Appointments

Date: _____   Gestational Age: _____   My Weight Gain: _____   Blood Pressure: _____

Other important & memorable events (baby's heartbeat, what doctor said, etc.):

_____

_____

_____

_____

Date: _____   Gestational Age: _____   My Weight Gain: _____   Blood Pressure: _____

Other important & memorable events (baby's heartbeat, what doctor said, etc.):

_____

_____

_____

_____

Date: _____   Gestational Age: _____   My Weight Gain: _____   Blood Pressure: _____

Other important & memorable events (baby's heartbeat, what doctor said, etc.):

_____

_____

_____

_____

Date: _____   Gestational Age: _____   My Weight Gain: _____   Blood Pressure: _____

Other important & memorable events (baby's heartbeat, what doctor said, etc.):

_____

_____

_____

_____

My Prenatal Appointments

Date: _____   Gestational Age: _____   My Weight Gain: _____   Blood Pressure: _____

Other important & memorable events (baby's heartbeat, what doctor said, etc.): _____

_____

_____

_____

Date: _____   Gestational Age: _____   My Weight Gain: _____   Blood Pressure: _____

Other important & memorable events (baby's heartbeat, what doctor said, etc.): _____

_____

_____

_____

Date: _____   Gestational Age: _____   My Weight Gain: _____   Blood Pressure: _____

Other important & memorable events (baby's heartbeat, what doctor said, etc.): _____

_____

_____

_____

Date: _____   Gestational Age: _____   My Weight Gain: _____   Blood Pressure: _____

Other important & memorable events (baby's heartbeat, what doctor said, etc.): _____

_____

_____

_____

My Prenatal Appointments

Date: _____   Gestational Age: _____   My Weight Gain: _____   Blood Pressure: _____

Other important & memorable events (baby's heartbeat, what doctor said, etc.):

_____

_____

_____

_____

Date: _____   Gestational Age: _____   My Weight Gain: _____   Blood Pressure: _____

Other important & memorable events (baby's heartbeat, what doctor said, etc.):

_____

_____

_____

_____

Date: _____   Gestational Age: _____   My Weight Gain: _____   Blood Pressure: _____

Other important & memorable events (baby's heartbeat, what doctor said, etc.):

_____

_____

_____

_____

Date: _____   Gestational Age: _____   My Weight Gain: _____   Blood Pressure: _____

Other important & memorable events (baby's heartbeat, what doctor said, etc.):

_____

_____

_____

My Sonogram Photos

My Fetal Movements Tracking Chart

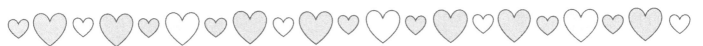

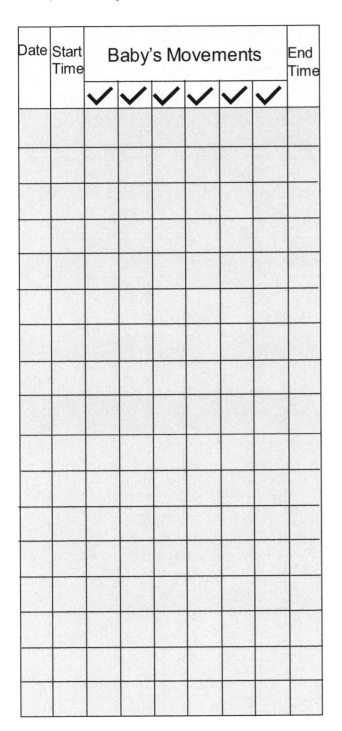

Date	Start Time	Baby's Movements						End Time
		✓	✓	✓	✓	✓	✓	

Date	Start Time	Baby's Movements						End Time
		✓	✓	✓	✓	✓	✓	

Important: Be sure to speak to your doctor or midwife to find out when and how to count your baby's movements.

My Fetal Movements Tracking Chart

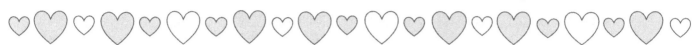

Date	Start Time	Baby's Movements						End Time
		✓	✓	✓	✓	✓	✓	

Date	Start Time	Baby's Movements						End Time
		✓	✓	✓	✓	✓	✓	

Important: Be sure to speak to your doctor or midwife to find out when and how to count your baby's movements.

My Fetal Movements Tracking Chart

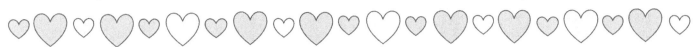

Date	Start Time	Baby's Movements						End Time
		✔	✔	✔	✔	✔	✔	

Date	Start Time	Baby's Movements						End Time
		✔	✔	✔	✔	✔	✔	

Important: Be sure to speak to your doctor or midwife to find out when and how to count your baby's movements.

My Favorite Pregnancy & Baby Resources

Pregnancy & Baby Books: _____

_____

_____

_____

_____

_____

_____

_____

_____

Websites: _____

_____

_____

_____

_____

_____

_____

_____

_____

_____

_____

_____

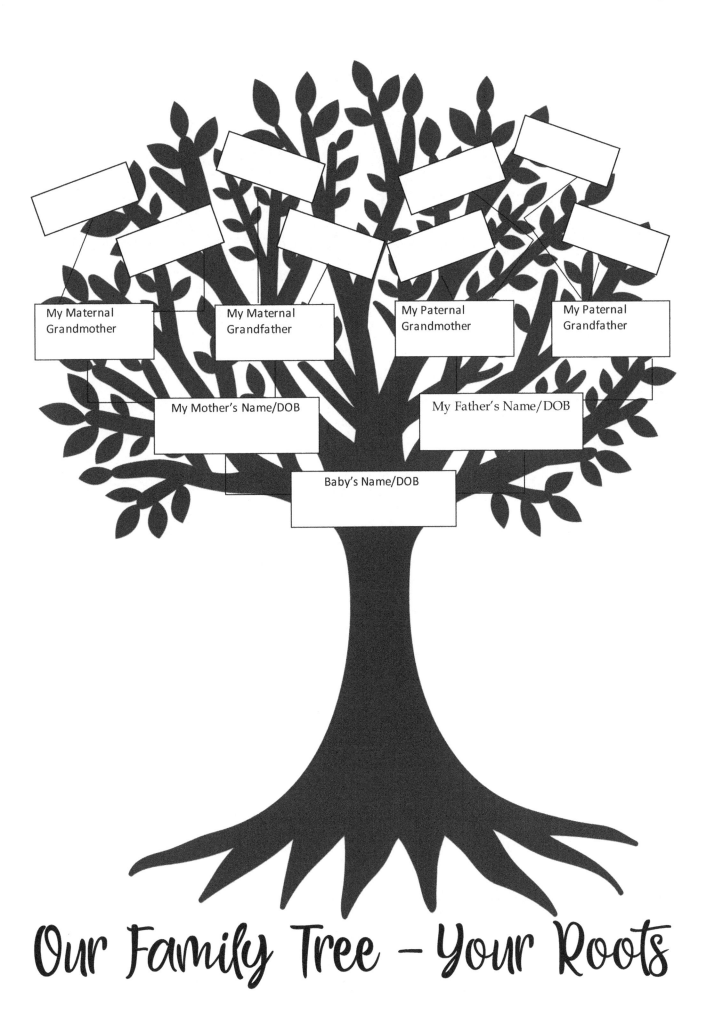

My Maternal Grandmother

My Maternal Grandfather

My Paternal Grandmother

My Paternal Grandfather

My Mother's Name/DOB

My Father's Name/DOB

Baby's Name/DOB

Our Family Tree – Your Roots

Create your own family tree from scratch if you need to represent divorces or deaths, and resulting remarriages that may have occurred in your family.

Baby's full name/DOB

Exercise During Pregnancy

Questions to ask my doctor or midwife & his/her responses:

(Keep in mind that some responses may vary depending on what trimester of pregnancy you're in and what is going on with you medically so be sure to revisit these questions with your doctor throughout your pregnancy)

Is it safe to exercise during my pregnancy?

Are there any risks of exercising while I'm pregnant?

What precautions should I take during exercise?

How much exercise should I get?

What are the best cardio and strength exercises I can do when I'm pregnant?

What exercises should I avoid during pregnancy?

What are warning signs that indicate I should stop exercising?

Names of Reputable Pregnancy & Exercise Websites:

Important Pre-Birth Questions

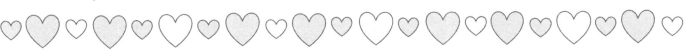

Do I want a midwife or obstetrician or my family doctor caring for me during my pregnancy, and why am I choosing one over the other?

What values are important to me when choosing my midwife or obstetrician (i.e. belief in natural process, breastfeeding knowledge, etc.)?

Is cord blood banking something we want to consider, and if so, where can we learn more?

If we have a boy, what are our thoughts on circumcision, and the risks and benefits?

Post more of your questions below:

My Birth Plan

Who I want present at the birth: _____

_____

My preferences for pain control: _____

_____

_____

My preferences re: medical interventions during labor: _____

_____

My preferences for medical interventions during delivery: _____

_____

_____

Who will cut the umbilical cord: _____

How I plan to feed my baby after birth: _____

_____

Most important issues to me: _____

_____

_____

Other: _____

_____

_____

_____

_____

Maternity Hospital Bag Checklist

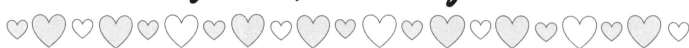

⭐ For Mom

- Medical cards & insurance documents
- Birth plan
- Lip balm
- Maternity or loose-fitting pants & top
- Socks & Slippers
- Nightgown & robe
- Nursing pillow
- Massage oil or lotion
- Panties
- Nursing bras
- Nipple cream
- Toothbrush, toothpaste, & floss
- Hair brush
- Shampoo & conditioner
- Skin care & cosmetics
- Sheets for crib
- Deodorant/antiperspirants
- Glasses, contacts, solution
-
-
-

⭐ For Birth Partner

- Snacks & water
- Phone, camera, video camera, & chargers
- Glasses & contact lens case
- Toothbrush & toothpaste
- Deodorant
- Change of clothes
- Book
- Money/credit card
-
-
-
-

⭐ For Baby

- Nightgown
- Sleepers
- Car seat
- Going-home outfit
- Socks & slippers
- Outerwear appropriate for the season
- Receiving blankets
- Pacifier
-
-
-
-
-

The Birth

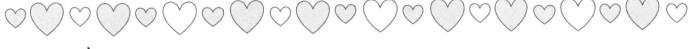

Baby's Full Name: _____

WELCOME TO THE WORLD!

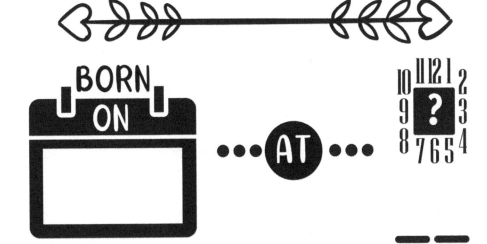

BORN ON

AT

WEIGHING & MEASURING

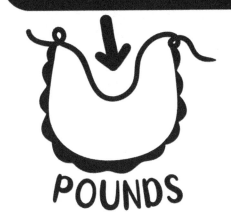

POUNDS

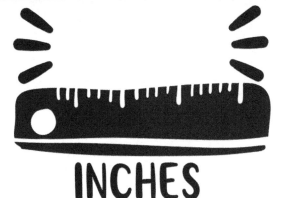

INCHES

Made in the USA
Columbia, SC
18 March 2020